HOW TO BEAT THE
WEIGHT LOSS
BLUES

A Definitive Guide to Long Term Weight Loss
Researched and Written by Jim Cabeceiras

authorHOUSE®

AuthorHouse™
1663 Liberty Drive
Bloomington, IN 47403
www.authorhouse.com
Phone: 1 (800) 839-8640

Published by AuthorHouse   08/30/2016

ISBN: 978-1-5246-2389-0 (sc)
ISBN: 978-1-5246-2388-3 (e)

Library of Congress Control Number: 2016913071

Print information available on the last page.

This book is printed on acid-free paper.

Important note: Consult with a physician before beginning a weight loss or exercise program.

CONTENTS

INTRODUCTION

Before you begin to conquer your challenges with weight loss, it's important to understand and accept the existence of two universal principles, or conditions. They are vital for your success. The first condition has nothing to do with will power, food choices, or counting calories, and everything to do with your ability to accept a new definition of success.

Success, relative to weight loss, is defined as the ability to reach an ideal goal weight and maintain an ideal weight for a minimum of three years. Reaching a thirty day weight loss goal, within the framework of this definition, is a successful action, but the result, whether it was a loss of five or ten pounds, generates a false feeling of achievement. Why? In truth, you still own a set of harmful eating triggers, and the eating habits you have created through these triggers are too powerful to overcome in thirty days. The problem is - you and I are programmed to think in terms of 'willing' our way to lost pounds over a fixed number of days or weeks, and once achieved, all the sabotaging demons in our heads will disappear. But they don't! This belief continues to be reinforced in the marketplace, leaving most of us perplexed and frustrated. With all the media hype and propaganda on weight loss, you need to know how to separate fact from fiction. You need a personal roadmap to success. This new approach has little to do with your chosen diet plan, and everything to do with learning how to control your emotional, instinctual, and biological drive to eat. Moving forward, you must accept this new definition of success as your own personal standard.

Second, you need to recognize your tendency to gain weight as a natural process, and purge your mind of the negative label you may be placing on yourself. You are not and never will be a failure when it comes to managing your weight. We are all programmed to measure our personal achievements in terms of 'success or failure', without margin for error, but this mindset will never apply to weight management. Weight gain is a natural and expected outcome in modern times, so beating yourself up over your current lack of control is self-defeating. Look at your pathway to success as a twisting, turning road with constant detours and distractions. It's important to remain focused on your final destination, and look at off road events (occasions when you over-indulge) as part of the process. Accept the fact that your path to salvation will never be a straight line. Removing feelings of guilt will help you move forward with confidence and maintain a positive frame of mind.

With a new definition of success in mind, it becomes critical for you to accept a new approach to losing weight – ***a back door approach*** – one rarely discussed in the media, but a path offering the absolute highest degree of success. It's termed a 'back door' approach because the information you need to access exists in the back of your mind, so to speak. You need to discover things about yourself that ***cause*** you to feel the way you do about food and eating. If you can accomplish this, the source of all your harmful triggers and impulses become easy to identify. Once identified, triggers become easy to manage. Let's examine this highly successful approach, beginning with the physical brain, the mind, and the instincts within.

In terms of existence, relative to the brain and the non-physical mind, you and I exist in two separate states, or levels of consciousness. One is a ***conscious*** state, where brain neurons fire and senses are activated, controlling speech, sight, physical movement, and our unique ability to reason. The second state of existence, a more subtle and mysterious condition - is the ***subconscious.*** Imagine your subconscious mind as the 'driver behind the wheel' of all the conscious thoughts you have – every minute of every day. The role it plays is a very primitive one, and its general purpose is to keep you alive. Your drive for sex (to mate), to fight or flee, to seek shelter, and your primitive drive to eat are essential for human survival, and these drives have controlled our behavior and formed our habits from the beginning of our existence. Because survival instincts, relative to eating, are buried deep in the lower brain (the back of your mind), you have no choice but to live in a constant state of confrontation when it comes to managing your appetite. But, as you will discover, there are ways to diminish the influence of these instincts and gain much more control than you have now.

Two worlds of consciousness demand an approach to weight loss that identifies both domains, but, as you will learn, ***challenges with diet and exercise originate in the subconscious.*** Looking for ways to better manage eating instincts is not a widely used approach in weight loss, and for most, it's a rejected strategy because it conflicts with what you see and hear in the media. The truth is, without identifying the sabotaging effects of your lower brain, you will never free yourself from the 'weight loss blues'.

What is the best approach to facilitate long term weight loss? It's a process of education and application, where you identify your own personal set of challenges and learn how to manage them. A few of your eating triggers may appear easy to identify, but your ability to identify personal challenges is only part of your solution. You also need a plan. You need a plan that offers the highest degree of personal success. If you decide to use the step by step approach outlined in this book, you will uncover your own set of challenges and learn how to systematically overcome their influence. Even better, your success will last a lifetime! ***Establishing permanent control of your eating style is the only valid pathway to success.*** Managing your own set of barriers is the single best approach you can take to accomplish this. As you continue to read, you will understand more about your eating behavior, how to facilitate lasting change, and why, moving forward, you should never consider a short term weight loss plan.

Statistics show a 95% failure rate as a natural and expected outcome for the millions of Americans taking the standard approach. The reason: With few exceptions, weight loss companies emphasize food choices, calories, supplements, suppressants, and other superficial remedies, and place little or no focus on managing eating 'triggers' or creating new eating habits. With this back door approach, you reap the rewards of a plan offering simple, natural solutions that stand the test of time. No hype, no drugs, no threat to your health or well being, no grocery purchase plan, and best of all, no lifestyle overhaul!

Let's start with a brief education on human history and behavior. It's important to gain a clear understanding of the effect your ancestors have on your current thinking. With this working knowledge in place, it will become clear 'why' this back door approach is effective, why almost all diets and weight loss plans offer only the ***illusion*** of success, and why seventy percent of our population remain stuck in the 'weight loss blues' rut. The truth will surprise you, educate you, inspire you, and keep you on a path to success. Read on.

THE OBESITY EPIDEMIC (WHAT YOU NEED TO KNOW)

Without question, the world you live in has an influence on your eating habits. You and I are inter-connected through social, cultural, and family influences – guiding our thoughts and actions in all behaviors – including our approach to eating. You need to know what these influences are, why they exist, how they work against you, and finally, what you can do gain more control.

The History of Human Eating Behavior. Within the past fifty thousand years, the human race has evolved through three stages of food behavior. Early humans lived as nomadic wanderers, living off what they could find or kill, spending the majority of their daylight hours in a vigilant quest for food. As recently as five thousand years ago, however, our transformation into the 'farmer role' took center stage. Humans began to settle in one place. We grew our own crops and tended livestock, eliminating the need to wander and search for food, and dramatically decreased the threat of starvation. Within the past hundred years, however, we find ourselves in a third stage of evolution – one of industrialization, mass production, and convenience. Food is now inexpensive, accessible, and plentiful. *The problem is, you and I possess the same instinctive approach to eating as our nomadic ancestors.* Five thousand years is simply not enough time, on an evolutionary scale, to change the way we process survival instincts relative to food and eating behavior. Look at modern cultures over a tiny fraction of evolutionary time – the past fifty years - and you can see the destructive relationship of eating instincts in an environment where food is plentiful, cheap, and convenient. The result, of course, is the highest rate of obesity in our history! In only the past fifty years! And rates are climbing every year. To make matters worse, we live in an age of advanced technology, embracing the concept of less physical work, and this condition may be adding to the challenges you face in your own life. Seventy percent of all adult Americans are now classified as overweight, resulting in what is now a full-blown health epidemic with no apparent end in sight[1]. But, if this statistic is correct, then, what about the remaining thirty percent who are not overweight? It doesn't make sense, given we all share the same environment and the same DNA. Do they know something you don't? Not really. Here's the question you should be asking yourself: Is there a way to reverse my pattern of weight gain that won't overwhelm me and push me to return to old habits? The answers is… yes! First, the bad news. There is no single magic bullet 'method' to weight loss. The good news, however, is that you have a finite number of obstacles to overcome, and these personal barriers can be identified and managed successfully.

Like a fingerprint, you own a unique blend of triggers that identify you alone. As you read, you will recognize many of your challenges, but more importantly, you will discover a few hidden challenges that have held you back in the past. Again, for real success, you need to break down every roadblock to success if your intent is to reach an ideal weight and remain there. The truth is – ***with the information available in the marketplace, and the tools you have to work with today, you are not prepared for real success!***[2]

YOUR SUBCONSCIOUS 'BACK DOOR' CONNECTION

In the southern most part of your brain, you own a set of survival instincts. Think of them as the driver of all behavior – your primal desire for sex (finding a mate), the seeking of shelter, the impulse to fight or flee, the need to socialize, and, your instinctive desire to eat. Primitive eating instincts are the common denominator, influencing every decision you make regarding food choices and the development of your current eating style.

ANCIENT EATING BEHAVIORS AND MODERN CULTURE

For our nomadic ancestors, we know that food was scarce, competition for food was a life and death struggle, and starvation was a daily threat to survival. The effort to hunt, skin, and prepare a single meal was a collective social task, and these events dominated human behavior because they dominated most of our waking hours. Ancient humans were forced to develop food behaviors that had one common intention – avoid starvation! In simple terms, the 'instinctive baggage' you and I carry are survival behaviors, relative to eating, that are useless in modern times. These instincts served us well over the past fifty thousand years, but today, they are a liability, and they make weight loss virtually impossible (unless you know how to manage them!). Obesity is a natural course in modern times, and, rates are rising for this one, simple reason: *In America and other industrialized countries, our food environment has changed over the past one hundred years while instinctive and social eating behaviors remain unchanged.* Now that food is cheap, convenient, and plentiful, starvation is no longer a threat to survival for most of us. We have become less physical as well – both in work and play - and this influence makes modern life even more challenging. You need to know what drives you to eat more than you need and why the thought of exercising creates such a negative mindset. Otherwise, efforts to cut calories or begin an exercise program become personal battles between your 'power of will' and your instincts. Your subconscious never sleeps, so the destructive signals you experience flow endlessly into your conscious brain, while the strength of your conscious 'will power' fluctuates between moments of strength and moments of weakness. Moments of weakness are a given, so the subconscious, through tenacity alone, wins the battle of control. ***The use of will power, without other distractions – or substitutions – is not sustainable.*** The real 'solution' for a lifetime of success in managing your weight lies in your answer to this question: 'How do I change years of eating habits influenced by thousands of years of evolved eating instincts'? Again, if you look toward the media or subscribe to one of thousands of weight loss plans, you see a common diet message of: 'eat this, not that' and with exercise - 'do this, not that'. Are these approaches a path to salvation? Absolutely not! The problem is, you and I are conditioned to buy into this process and skip the most important step in successful weight management. Think about your answer to this question: If I remain uneducated and food addicted, how effective will a weight loss program be? How effective will stimulants or appetite suppressants be? The point is this: For weight loss success to take hold over the span of a lifetime, your first order of business is to identify and manage your own set of triggers. It's only when you get a handle on ***the cause of over-eating***, that you put yourself in a position to follow through, with success, on the diet or exercise plan of choice. ***The effort to manage personal triggers is the single most important step in an attempt to lose weight.*** You can't choose a diet plan and 'will power' your way to lasting success without going through this process! Again, most Americans fail (Polls show less than 2% make it past the third year) because eating triggers are completely unique for each of us, and these personal barriers to success are not being identified. ***This process defines the 'Back Door' approach, which***

is, to place your focus on managing eating triggers and the instincts behind them, instead of the methods used by the majority – that is – choosing a diet plan, using the 'white-knuckle will power' approach, and hoping for the best. In addition, you need to understand the concept of will power as it applies to appetite control. By definition, when you talk about confronting your drive to eat, will power is a conscious effort to resist the demands of your biological drive (physical hunger) and your subconscious drive (avoid starvation). It is not a trait, but rather a developed ability to manage the impulses of your lower brain – all your primitive instincts and emotions. We have laws that force us to control most of our impulses, but morality, ethics, religious doctrine, and acceptable social standards of conduct come into play as well. Most of us develop self control as children and continue the process into adulthood, but with food and eating behavior, there is no public scorn for weight gain or for bringing a batch of decadent brownies to the church social. Poor eating habits are socially acceptable by the majority, and this condition leaves many of us with little or no incentive to change. Not permanently, anyway. Those who struggle with weight gain experience feelings of confrontation and anxiety on a daily basis as they attempt to gain more control over eating impulses, and because no current authority or government entity can force anyone into a weight loss program (not yet, anyway), this 'coping' skill is underdeveloped. The common belief that will power is a trait we 'possess' is misleading, and holding on to this belief decreases your chance for long term success.

Adding to the challenge, if you tend to identify with the majority, your past failures often resulted in a shift of blame to the diet process itself, creating a mindset of: "That diet didn't work for me" or "Diets don't work". But the reality is, weight loss is sustainable over the long haul if you take your primary focus off food choices and begin to tame the 800 pound gorilla in your head.

The Social Connection. In our industrialized countries, where food is plentiful and accessible, cultures are 'food oriented' because food has been a valued commodity throughout our history, and this belief is still a powerful influence on attitudes today. As early as a few hundred years ago, food was used in trade, commonly as a form of barter. As a result, owning and controlling food commerce translated to high levels of social status and power. We still carry the burden of all these behaviors and beliefs today, though most of us have cheap and easy access to food sources. ***You and I are pre-wired to place an inflated value on food.*** To make matters worse, we are conditioned, from infancy, to over-eat and to make food choices based primarily on taste. As a result, the majority of food commerce today is a competition for foods with taste appeal, and this translates to inexpensive, high-fat, high sugar, and highly processed food alternatives. Oddly enough, in the United States, the segment of our population who live in poverty have the highest rate of obesity![3] However, if food abundance was a true sign of social status, shouldn't the wealthiest segment of our population have the highest rate of obesity? Obviously, food no longer has the value it once held. Bottom line - you and I continue to feel this influence, and this 'false feeling' has to be recognized and kept in check.

As a social animal, you face added challenges with your need to identify and gain acceptance in society - which means developing many of the same habits and behaviors. For most of us, these formed habits and behaviors work against our effort to manage and maintain a healthy weight.

DEFINING YOUR EATING INSTINCTS

At its core, your lower brain wants you to not only live, but thrive. It motivates your eating behavior with one recurring thought, and that is – ***avoid starvation!*** Biology plays a conscious role by sending signals to your brain when you are hungry, but the underlying fear of starvation is the dominant, relentless drive, originating in your subconscious mind and influencing your conscious eating behavior – all day, every day. This ancient drive controls your thinking through ***four instinctive demands.***

First, your subconscious reminds you to eat when food is in your immediate environment. The instinctive message coded in your brain is: 'When food is available – eat!' In the interest of survival, you have the urge to 'over-eat' today because tomorrow may bring famine. Your lower brain simply ignores the fact that you have cash on hand and the local deli is minutes away. It (the subconscious) demands overindulgence. The human race would be extinct if not for this coded behavior. It explains why the buffet table can be so hard to resist – even if you are not hungry! Whether it's by accident or through conscious effort, your skinny friends and family members are successfully managing this impulse. Obviously, being constantly bombarded with the drive to over-eat is destructive in today's environment.

Second, your subconscious commands you to 'over value' and reward with food. This instinct is another major liability in modern times. If you were to give or receive a box of candy, a basket of fruit, or a baked ham, is the intent to prevent starvation? Of course not! Not consciously, anyway. The problem is, we are all instinctively driven to place a high value on food and to use a reward system based on a social sense of community, where individuals cooperate with a group in an effort to avoid any potential threat of starvation. Today, our culture makes it easy for most of us to survive, yet the sense of 'community' effort in survival remains part of our instinctive makeup. Add the false belief that offering tasty treats make you a good provider, or that being generous with food proves how much you care for others, and you get a clear picture of just how destructive this thinking is. Consciously, you know starvation is no longer a threat. But your lower brain disagrees. To gain perspective on how strong this feeling is, imagine offering your neighbor a slice of bread as a gift. You would feel awkward and foolish - at best. However, when you dig into your subconscious, you see that your ancient brain, tapped into the mindset of a nomadic wanderer, is fine with the prospect of helping a neighbor avoid starvation.

Third, all humans are committed to habit, rejecting any form of change. Because eating offers instant pleasure without immediate pain, the concept of reducing or eliminating your favorite foods is rejected by the pleasure/pain dynamic in your subconscious. You are habitual by nature, so changing the eating habits you have now is much more confrontational than you might expect. Think of eating habits as a locomotive, starting off slow when you were young and gaining momentum as you age. Once ten years of eating patterns are established, changing direction becomes difficult. After twenty years, an attempt to change can be overwhelming. Most of us don't understand this subconscious dynamic and what needs to happen for real change to take place. You can't stop the train, but as you read on, you will learn how to alter your direction just enough to reverse the destructive course you may be on now.

Finally, as a social animal, your instincts command you to identify with a group, directing you to conform to a culture that is your worst enemy when it comes to eating behavior. We all want to fit in and become accepted by the people around us. You and I are, by nature, social animals. But you need to be aware of the destructive relationship of this condition with your eating habits. Remember, most of your family and friends have issues with weight management themselves (remember, seventy percent of our population is overweight). In your effort to conform, you have created a major roadblock to your own ability to manage your weight. This barrier – the strong desire you have to follow the same approach to eating as the majority – must be identified, understood, and managed. Otherwise, returning to old habits becomes a completely natural and expected event.

With these four primal instincts working against you, it's easy to understand why weight gain is a natural course for anyone living in modern times. Without a plan to manage their effect on you, daily attempts to cut calories fall short because your strength of will remains fragile - like a feather in the wind – at the mercy of your lower brain's agenda. Again, should you reject this approach, the changes you force upon yourself – purging your kitchen of junk food, joining the local gym, or enrolling in a weight loss program – end up as temporary fixes, offering a dismal success rate of only five percent in the first year.

These four instincts, combined with modern living, have created ten major challenges to weight management. Some are recognizable, but most are misunderstood. As you read, you will begin to understand the role they have played in your life. But even more important, you will discover what you can do to finally 'beat the weight loss blues'. Imagine the peace of mind you will feel when the act of restricting calories is no longer a source of daily stress and anxiety.

THE TEN BARRIERS TO WEIGHT LOSS SUCCESS
(AND HOW TO BREAK THEM DOWN)

Barrier One: Lack of Education. Knowledge is the number one barrier and the fundamental challenge for most of us – for two simple reasons. First, without a basic understanding of what drives your eating behavior, it won't matter how determined you are or what diet you choose to follow – you will have temporary success at best! You need to know what's behind the curtain – the unknown, primal forces that break you down. Once identified, you then need to be educated enough to know what strategies offer success and why the collective methods used today result in repeated frustration and failure.

The second reason - knowledge is power. If your goals and expectations of weight loss are based on facts, it becomes much easier to succeed. Americans spend over sixty billion dollars each year on weight loss products and services - books, DVD's, magazines, meal delivery services, and thousands of advertised plans that are predominantly worthless, and you need to be educated enough to know why. In addition, when you examine your initiative to learn, seeking the truth is a relatively minor challenge compared to the multiple barriers you face in your own struggle. *A half-hearted quest for knowledge indicates a half-hearted intent to lose weight.* Open your mind and accept new information. Put yourself in a position to achieve realistic weekly goals, so when you reach them you can gain confidence, and your desire to give up fades into a distant memory. The first item on your agenda is the purging of all weight loss and exercise propaganda you have been exposed to over the years. Replace the mythical and theoretical with factual information from scientific and medical sources. ***View all weight loss claims with a healthy dose of skepticism.*** But most important, as you continue to read, begin to identify and understand your own challenges. Even for the educated among us, an effort to shed pounds can feel like a climb up Mount Everest in a t-shirt and sandals.

Once you are empowered with knowledge, you have a foundation, and you put yourself in a position to manage food addiction and all other barriers blocking your path to success. Common beliefs you hold now – that are, in fact, myths - can be dispelled.

The 'Body Weight' Myth. This is a perfect example of a collective lack of knowledge. With few exceptions, the diet industry's marketing strategy of 'body weight' and 'body fat' being one in the same is misleading. The truth is, they are not. In fact, the process of losing body fat is an exact science and contradicts much of what is presented in the media. ***You must have a deficit of 3,500 calories in order to lose one pound of body fat***[4]. Take this number, write it in big black letters, and post it on your refrigerator – that's how important it is! Losing two pounds of body fat in a week requires a deficit of 7,000 calories. Can you handle a decrease of 1,000 calories a day? A reduction of 500 calories per day (one pound of body fat lost per week) is still good progress – and easier to maintain. Knowing these facts, do you think it's possible to lose five pounds of body fat in one week? That's 17,500 calories less, or 2,500 calories per day you need to burn or eliminate from your diet! Can you *really* lose five pounds in one week? Yes, you can. But the biology behind this condition is easily explained: The five pounds of 'weight' lost is a combination of body fat, lean tissue, water (fluid), and in many cases, waste emissions. The FDA estimates the average adult at 2,000 calories consumed per day [5], so, again, for the purpose of losing body fat, is a 2,500 daily calorie deficit even conceivable? Can you decrease your daily calories to 1,000 and use exercise to account for the other 1,500 calories? This would mean virtually starving yourself every day for one week and pulling off two-hour sessions of exercise - every day! You have to come to grips with this reality and ignore virtually all weight loss advertisements and media messages. The truth is - beginning a new, healthier diet typically decreases your sodium levels and increases your consumption of fiber. Sodium holds water and fiber increases regularity, so a loss of three pounds (or more) per week in the first few weeks can and should be expected. Again, body fat should be your only concern. Not the scale (Total Bodyweight), and not Body Mass Index (BMI). Keep it simple. ***Monitor your percentage of body fat, use a mirror and the fit of your clothing as primary feedback, and finally, use the scale as a secondary monitor of progress – once or twice per week!***

If you continue to reject biological facts or look for shortcuts, you doom yourself to repeated frustration, and that state of mind translates to multiple failed attempts at weight loss. ***What is a valid goal? In the real world, there is only one legitimate pace – one to two pounds of lost body fat per week. The loss of water, waste, or lean tissue is <u>not</u> legitimate weight loss!*** Cases of morbid obesity and some medical conditions may be exceptions to this rule, but for the majority, a 'one to two pounds per week' pace should be the goal of choice. Remember, you must have a deficit of 3,500 calories to lose one pound of body fat. Write down the phrase 'One to two pounds per week' and 'body fat is the only weight that counts' and post them in a conspicuous place. You may have to re-visit these universal truths time and again.

The bottom line is: Choosing to remain uneducated indicates your intent, which is to stay the way you are. You may believe you have a chance at success by subscribing to one of many national diet programs, but if the science of nutrition, fitness, and solutions to changing your future eating and exercise behaviors are not included in the plan, your investment will not reap permanent rewards. *Guidelines on what to eat and how to cook healthy alternatives are terrific tools, but the process of selecting, purchasing, cooking, and eating food is a conscious plan of action, and ignores 95% of your problem – overcoming the destructive instincts inside you. Without a 'Back Door' approach to weight loss, you set yourself up to fail.* Start with learning the basics – for example – how and why your subconscious plots against you when you attempt to make changes, and, what you can do to overcome this automatic rejection to change. Learn the process we all have to go through in order to diminish poor eating and exercising habits, and what form of action needs to be taken in order to establish new, healthier habits. Do you know how this process works? Can you establish new, healthier eating habits over a period of thirty days? Has a diet company's support team ever given you a valid solution to managing your addiction to food? If you know these answers, your chance of success increases exponentially. Reflect on what you see and hear in the media. With a little knowledge, you begin to see a predominantly hollow message. Without the foundation of an education, you set yourself up to lose the war on weight gain because you remain vulnerable to suggestion. Do you know how many calories you burn each day? Do you know what to look for on food labels? Do you know some basics facts about your metabolism? If you reach a point where you know the answers to these questions, you set yourself up to succeed. Keep this thought in mind - you can become the most inspired and self-determined individual on the planet, but without knowledge (specifically, knowing how to facilitate lasting change), you become a high performance sports car on the open road – with no direction or destination. The good news, for you, is that once you read and understand the solutions defined within the pages of this book, your education barrier all but disappears!

Barrier Two: Food Addiction. Food addiction, referred to as 'emotional eating' in the media, is an undisputable cause of weight gain. We (humans) have a tendency to seek food in almost all emotional situations - when bored, sad, anxious, angry, hurt, depressed, happy, seeking comfort (responding to stress), socializing, or pacifying the developed habit of eating when we have easy access to food (at home watching T.V., for example). All the experts are in agreement regarding the emotional attachment we all have to food. However, simply identifying the problem of addiction, as it relates to you, is meaningless. After years of daily repetition, can you simply stop eating your favorite foods or snacks? The answer is 'no'. You need a legitimate plan of action that addresses the fundamental question of: "How do I break the habit of eating when I am not hungry?" A natural and highly effective solution to food addiction does exist. The problem is, this knowledge is rarely discussed in the media or through the marketing efforts of our weight loss industry.

First, let's begin with the facts: ***Food addiction is both psychological and biological.*** In recent years, studies have found that when we indulge in tasty foods, chemical endorphins are released and attach to receptors within the brain[6]. Endorphins are 'feel-good', morphine chemicals manufactured by the body in response to pleasurable experiences and sensations, like eating your favorite foods. This challenge is compounded by the fact that your 'feel-good-food-fix' is temporary. The euphoria (blood sugar induced high) quickly dissipates and your search for pleasure in food sources begins again. The result, in today's world, with easy access to tasty foods, is significant weight gained through biological and behavioral conditioning! Addiction is an expected result when you examine your behavior, specifically, your subconscious desire to seek pleasure via endorphin release, avoid pain (the potential threat of starvation), and follow through on your lower brain instincts. Moving from one endorphin high to the next is a completely natural behavior. For this reason alone, eating habits become consistent over time. Modern commerce adds to your addiction challenges by offering cheap and instant access to processed and refined foods designed to appeal to taste – and loaded with calories. The solution, for you, involves another important human condition: ***Eating is not the only endorphin producing activity in your life.*** Is food indulgence your only pleasure in life? Of course not! Many of your hobbies, interests, and social activities produce identical endorphin highs. You have another advantage, too. These 'other' activities offer more sustained highs, lasting hours instead of minutes (the temporary dopamine high from a candy bar, for example). You can assume, from this condition, that in order to conquer food addiction, you must explore and expand other activities in your life that produce 'feel-good chemicals' in your brain. Exercise, participation in project or hobby you enjoy, working on career goals, family and social interplay – even sex - can fill the endorphin void (pain) you create when you cut back on calories. This form of substitution is the most effective method you can use to conquer the barrier of food addiction, unless your problem is severe, in that you self-medicate with food to the point of obesity and deeper emotional problems need to be addressed through counseling. This form of 'substitution therapy' works because you pro-actively replace the emotional and biological void (pain) created by denying yourself the pleasure offered by your favorite foods. Remember, your subconscious works hard to maximize pleasure and minimize pain, so when you limit the foods you enjoy, you upset this balance. Your past eating habits become a beckoning siren, luring you back to the land of pleasure through the subconscious. The power of your will takes a back seat to this subconscious drive for instant pleasure. Food addiction is and will always be a completely natural course in today's culture, so your first order of business is to stop beating yourself up over your own lack of control.

Successfully managing addictive food behavior is a simple two-step process. First, you identify and understand this process in yourself (which you have now accomplished), and second, you must make a few bold lifestyle choices and act on them. Make a list of your 'top ten' activities (or interests) that have no connection with food or eating. Begin to make small changes by intentionally expanding the role of these interests. The truth about the relationship between food addiction and your inability to lose weight is this: ***Diets do not fail because of food addiction. Nature dictates a return to old habits when the emotional and biological void (pain) created by restricting calories is not replaced. If you 'substitute' other endorphin-producing activities, while keeping the restrictions in your diet to a minimum, you can successfully manage addictive eating.*** You must decide, before day one of your diet, to seek out and expand other activities and events in your life that create the same endorphin high. It may sound like the obvious solution now that you know the facts, but for the majority of Americans, brainwashed by a media selling superficial remedies, this form of 'addiction management' is either rejected or simply left out of the discussion. Rejection, in this case, is denial, because the comfort of food and the endorphin rush provided by eating may have helped our nomadic ancestors survive, but in today's environment, confronting the 800 pound gorilla in your head has become an absolute necessity.

The single best form of endorphin substitution is exercise, because it burns added calories and improves health (a triple benefit when you add the sustained endorphin high!). ***Denying yourself the same foods you have enjoyed in the past is a source of pain, and this pain will never be dominated by will power alone. Conscious efforts are always at the mercy of your subconscious drive to avoid the perceived pain of change.*** Expand other life passions, especially if they involve physical activity. If 'eating, snacking, and a sedentary lifestyle that includes hours of daily television and/or social media' describe your current lifestyle, food addiction is more than likely a barrier to your success. Subtle changes are absolutely necessary. In the first few weeks, it may feel uncomfortable to forgo a serving of ice cream, spend more time in the garden, become consistent with an exercise program, or simply expand other interests. However, like any other activity repeated consistently over time, it gains momentum and becomes accepted by your subconscious. Subtle, forced changes today become habits tomorrow. Food begins to play more of a 'sustenance role' instead of a common source of daily gratification and pleasure. This form of therapy is *the* fundamental solution to the problem of food addiction. Keep this thought in mind - you can take food out of your environment, but it will not change your desire for the endorphin rush food provides. If you can successfully manage a few minor changes that distract you from your focus on food gratification and commit to these changes for a minimum of six months, addictive food behaviors will have less influence on you. There is one undeniable truth: ***You will never eliminate your addiction to food.*** Your 'strength of will' fluctuates between periods of strength and weakness for the simple reason that biologically driven decisions to eat are never purely biological. There is always an emotional connection. But there is good news. A major lifestyle overhaul is not necessary. Completely eliminating your favorite foods is not a valid approach. Subtle changes, like two servings of ice cream per week instead of five, and spending a little more time on other endorphin producing activities are enough to minimize your addiction and reverse your pattern of weight gain. If you commit to this two step solution for six months, this major barrier will be reduced to where it needs to be – an occasional detour on your path to success.

Barrier Three: Resistance Skills. It's important to recognize another important human condition, that is - the ability to control eating impulses is a legitimate coping skill that can be improved over time. You and I are programmed to search for immediate remedies that require little effort and even less sacrifice - fad diets, quick weight loss schemes, drugs, stimulants, laxatives, or even surgical alternatives. But once you gain an understanding of how habits develop over time, you can begin to alter many of the poor eating habits you have now. ***To be skilled in any discipline, you have to practice through repetition, and the development of new, healthier eating habits is no different. Bottom line – food denial is a learned discipline!*** There has to be a commitment to practice new skills for more than just a week or a month at a time. If you think you can play the guitar like Eric Clapton after thirty days of practice, you join the majority of Americans, failing over and over again on their attempts to lose weight. Why? Because thirty days of effort may translate into a hundred daily 'challenges' in impulse control, but, in order to alter your behavior at the subconscious level, you need more experience. Accept the fact that it may take six months to a year to become a professional – that is – someone with above average coping skills. The fact is, your ability to restrict calories and make healthier food choices is a learned discipline. Your skill level may be under-developed now, but the good news is – you can always improve! The tiny fraction of our human population that manage to lose weight and keep it off for more than three years (less than 2%) have a developed resistance when it comes to daily eating behavior. This small minority of super-achievers have the same cravings and instincts as you and I, but they have better coping skills because they passed on the supersize and desert menus so many times, eating smaller meals and skipping desert no longer 'feel' like denial (pain). This evolved process actually works! The problem is – this 'practice' is rarely discussed or even presented in the media as a legitimate form of weight management. But the fact remains – it's a critical part of your solution! If you turn to food in times of stress, or have emotional attachments to food, these developed coping skills are an absolute necessity for success. Accept this concept: ***Forcing a new behavior to become part of your daily life, like the sacrifice of restricting calories, is a developed skill!*** If you can manage a consistent, successful effort for six months, you discover, in the sixth month, your once elevated levels of daily anxiety and pain are a fraction of what they used to be. Why? Of course, the answer is; the more skilled you become, the more the task becomes second nature, and the less you are influenced by your past behaviors (think of the process we all go through when we learn to drive a car). The result is – less emotional conflict and anxiety – and a high probability this new behavior will become your habit of choice. In simple terms, the more time you invest in consciously controlling your diet, the better you become at managing daily cravings and impulses. Again, the small, conscious changes you make today eventually migrate into your subconscious as newly formed habits. The transfer will never take place in thirty days, and the new habits you form will never dominate your lower brain's agenda. However, for most of us, this is good news. Why? Because a change in direction - where weight gain becomes weight loss - is a difference of less than three hundred calories per day! The smaller the change, the more likely it will bypass the automatic resistance of your subconscious and evolve into a lasting habit. Remember – it's in your nature to resist change! Even when a change in lifestyle is positive, and you consciously believe the change will benefit you, your subconscious will resist. Habits develop and create a personal comfort level in all of us. When you add the influence of this condition to your primal needs to satisfy hunger (avoid starvation), gorge yourself when food is abundant, maintain past eating habits, and identify with a culture of indulgence, you understand why your past attempts at weight loss were so difficult. ***Bottom line, these instincts are part of your subconscious resistance, and they will never be dominated by will power alone! To overcome them, you must commit to making small changes over an extended period of time – typically, six months to one year.*** Try a daily reduction of three to four hundred calories, combined with moderate exercise once or twice each week. You can accomplish this with little resistance from your lower brain and manage your social agenda as well. Once in place, it becomes much easier for you to maintain this new lifestyle for years. The fact is, without these incremental changes, the effort to restrict calories cannot be maintained because feelings of accomplishment and pleasure are outweighed by feelings of pain – eliminating calories, eating 'bland' food choices instead of your favorite foods, or missing out on the other emotional and social connections you have with food. However, if you could still eat many of your favorite foods and maintain most of your social eating habits, you would be more likely to repeat this process to a point in time when your new eating style becomes a habit of choice. This 'back door' approach to managing your weight is absolutely essential. Fact is, you will never completely eliminate poor eating choices, but you can decrease the frequency of poor choices by making subtle changes and setting simple, structured weekly goals that allow for a few indulgences. ***The reality is this: If you can see it, smell it, or know that it exists in your kitchen, you want it!*** Your environment, with all its food conveniences, demands that you become 'skilled' and establish better coping skills than you have now. Remember, there is no need to be completely resistant to the buffet table at the next social gathering. You just need more resistance than you have now. Understand and accept this concept: ***Small daily sacrifices (fewer calories) are meaningless if not repeated over several months. Coping skills eventually become more advanced and the stress of dieting decreases, but this process can take well over six months for some, and well over a year for others.*** If you can't muster up the patience to handle this commitment of time, or if you reject the concept of developing resistance skills, you are destined for a lifetime of on-and-off dieting, frustration, despair, and, eventually, a sub-standard quality of life. Contrary to what you hear from media experts, habits related to appetite cannot be eliminated or managed successfully within thirty days. Keep reading and you will understand why. To gain perspective, think of your daily effort to cut calories this way: 'Repeating a new, forced sacrifice one hundred times makes me an amateur. Repeating it one thousand times makes me a pro'. Your weight loss mantra should be; 'However long it takes'.

Barrier Four: Inability To Manage Stress. Stress is a diet killer, contributing to mental and physiological barriers including adrenaline overproduction, increases in stress hormone levels, a depressed immune system, mood swings, anxiety, depression, and lack of sleep[7]. Fatigue often contributes to unhealthy cravings for calorie-rich foods in an attempt to gain energy, leading to even more weight gain. In addition, your instinctive drive to eat contributes to personal stress levels when you restrict the foods you enjoy. In short, stress is a negative trigger for most of us in our relationship with food. With the endorphin rush provided through the consumption of your favorite foods, you can understand why the act of indulging in tasty foods and treats is a completely natural response to stress. *When personal levels of stress are high, seeking comfort in food is a natural response. This condition will not change. You are not a failure (though you may feel like one) when you turn to food for relief.* You are, in fact, just being human. The 'white-knuckle' will power approach has a tendency to fail during stressful times because of your instinct to seek comfort, and, because food offers both a psychological and biological feeling of well-being, it becomes a natural, easy outlet for managing stress. What you can do, however, is learn how to manage and diminish your own level of stress. And to be successful in managing stress, you have to understand its origin.

In simple terms, stress is the result of what you perceive as a threat or source of pain – both emotionally and physically.

There is always a cause and effect – experiences occur - and you react through conflicted, negative emotions - including rage, anxiety, sorrow, frustration, desperation, jealousy, disappointment, hostility, depression, and fear. Emotional pain causes physical changes as well, breaking down your health from the inside. All humans experience stress, but some of us appear to have a unique ability to maintain control over our state of mind and lead a much more blissful existence.

At the source, stress is about control, or lack thereof. But what would we like to control? Other people? Of course. Events? Yes. Relationships cause stress for the simple reason that the behavior of others cannot be controlled. Events cause stress because life can't be controlled, and life will always offer the element of surprise – good and bad. It's how you react to events and behaviors - the uncontrollable part of your life – that determine your level of personal stress. You can't control death, sickness, accidents, and most of your environment, so when unplanned events occur, stress levels tend to become elevated. When the event ends, stress levels fade. But stress affects some of us more than others, and the reason for this is very simple. We all live in two separate domains – the world we have control of and a world we will never control – but many of us have trouble understanding and identifying the differences. When you blur the lines between the two, stress levels tend to remain high. To lower your own level of daily stress, two things have to occur. First, you must understand the two domains of control and recognize your own 'imbalances'. You cannot invest yourself emotionally in what cannot be controlled. The end result of knowing and accepting the difference results in an *emotional balance*, which is critical in keeping your stress level in check. Second, you must learn how to relax and re-charge with ***downtime.*** These two lifestyle changes must become part of your own plan if your intent is to break free from stress-related eating.

Let's clarify the two domains of control even further. Your boss's foul moods, bad drivers, conflict in a relationship, or anything that sparks a negative emotional reaction in you – are in the non-control domain. How do you typically respond to these events? Once you identify these two domains, you can take steps to break down this barrier and take your stress down a notch. Then, if you can add some downtime into your life, stress levels will fall even further. ***You must take ownership of what you can control (food choices, for example) - but even more important, you have to gain more control over your reactions to the uncontrollable side of life.*** Levels of denial and irrational thinking begin to fade away when you can see, in your mind's eye, the distinct border between the two domains of control. When this happens, your ability to organize and manage your daily life improves. Your ability to sleep improves. You stop shifting blame away from yourself, so a 'victim mentality' (blaming others for your own shortcomings) will begin to disappear, too. Improved quality of sleep is a major beneficiary of lower stress, which, in turn, produces an improved ability to handle stress during your waking hours. Quality and quantity of sleep are essential! Lack of sleep is often linked to stress, and, with successful weight loss, many weight-induced sleep disorders disappear[8]. The stress barrier is not a difficult challenge when you understand where it comes from, but you need to take intentional steps that may feel awkward in the beginning.

First, understand the two worlds of control and decide you no longer want to be an emotional slave. Control what you can and forget about the rest. Then, set aside some downtime, or simply perform an activity you enjoy (other than eating) that alters your mood for the better. Try meditation, yoga, walking, massage, exercise, and surrounding yourself with people and environments that bring you peace of mind, or anything that allows you to escape, clear your head, and recharge. ***Remember this important condition: Restricting calories is a source of both emotional and physical stress! In order to remain focused on your diet, other stress influences have to be minimized.*** Periods of high stress make it almost impossible to maintain your diet – so don't! Focus on reducing stress to the point where you can re-gain control of your eating impulses again. DON'T TRY TO BE SUPERHUMAN! If you have stress related eating triggers, you have some work to do before you can begin a structured weight loss plan. Stress can and will dominate your life on occasion. You should expect occasional setbacks. Seek counseling if your stress levels are chronic or overwhelming.

A wise man once said: "Life is 10% what happens, and 90% how you react to it". If you can stop 'reacting' and start 'accepting' your inability to control people and events in your life, your stress levels will fall, the allure of your favorite comfort foods will fade, and you become emotionally equipped to handle the long term process of changing your eating style.

Barrier Five: Obsessing Over the Diet. Here's what you need to know for long term success: The concept of perfection does not exist in the world of weight loss. If you are a 'perfectionist' or tend to obsess over daily results, you set yourself up for a world of pain when it comes to weight loss - for one simple reason: ***Human nature cannot be denied! You <u>will</u> stray from your diet plan! It's not a matter of 'if', but 'when' you will indulge. If you reject this condition, your first 'cheating event' becomes a trigger, breaking down your confidence with conflicted and negative affirmations of failure. When this occurs, your drive to return to old habits becomes overwhelming.***

Be decisive about being 'on' or 'off' your diet, so when you eat for pleasure, you can enjoy the experience and move on. As I mentioned before, feeling like a failure or experiencing emotions of self-hatred are unwarranted and unjustified. If you manage to keep most of your meals and snacks in check throughout the week, you discover that a few poor choices may have slowed your progress, but, the reality was, you made progress. Taking an obsessive approach to weight loss, without a margin for error, puts you in a fragile emotional state - where your confidence is easily shaken and self-sabotage is eminent. Remember this fact - your strength of will is always dominated by your inner voice telling you to 'eat when food is available', 'follow the crowd', 'over-value food', and 'stick to habits of the past'. Bottom line, you need to purge the concept of 'cheating' when it comes to straying from your diet plan. Cheating implies guilt, and feeling guilty about being human is self-destructive. National experts and trainers talk of 'cheat meals' or 'cheat days', but the context is wrong! You should never feel guilty about being human. Plan to go off track, enjoy the moment, chalk it up as one of life's pleasures, and move on without the side order of guilt. If you are obsessive by nature, this can be a tough challenge. To break through this barrier, you simply need to accomplish two things.

First – stop micromanaging your diet! Give yourself a break from the fixation or obsession with foods and calories. Keeping a daily diary, measuring foods, standing on the scale every twelve hours, or making food the topic of conversation is destructive for the majority of dieters. Most of us can remember what we have eaten and estimate a fairly accurate daily total of calories consumed. A small investment in education will give you the tools you need. The reality is, the more you think about, write about, and talk about food and eating, the more it will dominate your thoughts. When this happens, you intentionally choose to battle with your instincts, and the more time you invest in direct confrontation with the demands of your subconscious, the higher your chance of failure becomes. Detach yourself from a constant fixation on planning, discussing, cooking, and preparing food. Use the food addiction solution (Barrier 2) of ramping up other activities that have little to do with food or the act of eating.

Second, you need to establish a new weekly goal that allows for kinks in your armor. Try this highly effective mindset: *'My Success this week will be defined by seventeen moderate, healthy meals (total of 21), and four opportunities to eat what I enjoy'*. This accomplishes two things. It removes feelings of guilt from your weekly agenda, and, because you can still enjoy most of your social and family obligations and the foods that come with them, you can carry on with your diet without feeling the emotional pain of isolation and social separation. In the world of weight loss, eating healthy, low calorie food choices for eight out of ten meals is, in fact, a recipe for success.

Let's dig a little deeper into why an obsessive, analytical approach to weight loss is often ineffective. When you examine the science behind weight loss, you see that the human body undergoes a constant barrage of influences that have subtle effects on weight and little to do with body fat. Changing hormone levels, sodium intake, physical and emotional stress, medications – even medical conditions - can have daily effects on your total weight, causing both gains and losses by as much as 2-3 pounds (mostly water) in less than twenty four hours[9]. It's possible to have a daily deficit of calories and still gain weight! Ouch! Bottom line, if you monitor your weight too closely, you will be disappointed, especially if you are allowing for a few indulgences each week. Stop the twice daily 'weigh-ins' (once or twice weekly is enough), and, stop beating yourself up over the fact that you enjoy an occasional cheeseburger or serving of ice cream. In other words, lighten up, stop micromanaging, and accept your human side. ***Remember, feelings of guilt and failure may be present in other areas of your life, but they do not apply to an effort to lose weight***. They never will. Weight gain is a natural course when you examine the instincts you were born with, the environment you live in, and the eating habits you have developed over the years. Failure in the dieting process is a given, so you have to accept the fact that setbacks will always be part of your new eating style. If you understand and accept this condition, a decadent lunch with friends won't chip away at your self-esteem with images of another glaring failure. Keep this thought in mind – a successful outcome is defined by your ability to reach an ideal weight and remain there. But you have to change your thinking from 'How fast can I get there?' to 'How do I get there...

and stay there?' Again, once you understand the inner workings of your lower brain and a few simple concepts in biology, you stop buying into the industry's 'faster is better' approach. If you can concede the fact that your path to weight loss success will never be void of trips and falls, you can maintain a positive frame of mind, day after day, and the frustration and despair you felt in the past will fade away.

Barrier Six: Isolation. Losing weight is a deeply personal struggle, and because food is associated with affection, gratitude, and social reward, choosing a restricted eating style can result in feelings of both social separation and isolation. For you, a 'me against the world' mentality can be a painful emotional stance because it conflicts with your desire to conform and identify. To add to your misery, this need becomes a burden if most of your friends and family are carrying a few extra pounds and have little or no desire to join you in your quest. The fact is, for most men and women, a few added pounds rarely generate feelings of embarrassment or confrontation. Why? Because thirty pounds of extra weight is not only socially acceptable today, but normal! *You must manage your instinctive need to identify with others as a potential barrier to long term weight loss.* A common trait successful dieters share is a sense of independence and self-belief – a valued asset when dealing with a new behavior that breaks away from the status quo. People who succeed long-term understand that not everyone will embrace and support a lifestyle that contradicts most of society, but they push forward anyway. *The truth is, you will be disappointed if you expect wholesale support of your new eating lifestyle.* Be prepared for a dose of passive aggressive resistance when you choose to stop identifying with the social food component of family and friends. The comment of 'One piece of pie won't kill you' really means, 'Why can't you be like the rest of us and be happy with a few extra pounds?' If you live with an uncooperative spouse, partner, or other family members, you should expect only small amounts of support. All social groups reject change, and changes in eating style are perceived as a threat to the group you seek approval and acceptance of. It becomes more personal when you reject your own past, where your parents, out of love, may have provided you with tasty foods and snacks, void of nutritional value, all without knowing just how harmful this pattern of eating would become. Rejecting what your family believes when it comes to food behavior can feel confrontational. But you need to understand this – the 'betrayal' you feel has little to do with your family's affection for you and everything to do with their lack of understanding – that there is no correlation between love and spoiling you with constant food gratification. You need to understand this behavior so you can recognize your negative feelings of isolation and betrayal as false emotions. Keep this thought in mind - your family and friends are simply feeling threatened (pain) when you fail to join in any form of collective indulgence. A social agenda that often involves food (dinners, birthdays, cookouts, family gatherings, parties, etc.) can be used as an opportunity to indulge in moderation, but identifying with an overweight majority is, in itself, a form of self-sabotage. *It won't matter how much determination you have, or how well you manage other personal triggers. If you can't break away from the social influences on your eating style, any success you achieve will be temporary.* Many of your overweight friends and family are enablers, and because weight loss is such a personal challenge, the odds are stacked against you as a social animal with an instinctive need to identify with the very people who are enabling you. When it comes to managing a new eating lifestyle, a structured support system can help, but you must evolve and become independent, like a teenager leaving the comfort of home and making their own way in the world. It is unreasonable to expect dependency to last! Eventually, you face this reality: 'I am on my own, managing impulses and poor habits without twenty-four hour support'. For long term success, your thought process has to become self-centered and self-reliant. You have to examine your intentions and goals, as well as your commitment to face down and break through your own set of barriers. Your need to identify, your expectations of emotional support, and your desire to gain acceptance must all be diminished. Again, diet plans that include counseling or group therapy are often effective, but they fail (over 95% of the time) as a long term solution because support, via one-on-one or group counseling, rarely uncover the specific set of challenges you alone possess. The truth is, for all adults, ***dieting is a personal challenge, not a shared responsibility***. It never will be. If you see it any other way, you doom yourself to failure because you expect consistent support, or worse, you feel justified in shifting a portion of blame or credit away from yourself. Weight loss, when successful, is a selfish, personal endeavor where the decision to sacrifice has little to do with group influence, a desire for acceptance, or a need to impress others. Be prepared to handle social situations, and take full responsibility for your eating habits, regardless of the situation. Case in point - if you join a group of friends for lunch, and they choose burgers and fries while you defiantly stick to your salad choice, where is the support? Who deserves the blame if you give in? When you experience this common social scenario, and you always will, it becomes critical for your own success to understand that the expectation of support is counter-productive (unless everyone you come in contact with is also dieting!). And, shifting blame is a one-way path to failure. When support is offered, accept and appreciate it, but understand that many of your friends, family, and co-workers will not identify with your new eating style. Remember, you and I are social animals, so breaking from the pack with eating behavior is subconsciously unacceptable to others. If you understand this condition, and, in addition, manage your destructive emotional need to shift blame away from yourself, you can successfully break through this barrier. Again, it's a back door approach, where you understand why you feel the way you do, and by answering the 'why' question, you stack the odds in your favor. But there are other questions you must answer: Do you have enough belief in yourself to handle a lack of support? Can you ignore a dose of passive-aggressive influence? Will you take full responsibility for your current condition? Can you emotionally align yourself with only those who support your effort? If you can accomplish these tasks, this barrier breaks down and widens your path to success.

Overcoming feelings of isolation and separation is a two-step process. The first step is acceptance: Don't let the 'non-dieters' get to you! Remember - providing tasty foods and snacks does not indicate love or affection for others! However, this perceived feeling, born thousands of years ago, is still part of your emotional make-up. Your loved ones still love you, but their primitive brain is in control – and sending the wrong message. You need to understand this condition so your own feelings of isolation and self-doubt can be kept in check. If you continue to feel 'left out' socially because you stopped participating in food indulgences, you will have a problem with maintaining a weight loss plan. For success, you have to understand your need to fit in, and separate your 'social eating desires' from the rest of your social life. *The second step involves a clear understanding of your nature to identify:* Don't fight your desire to be part of a group – use it to your advantage! Why not seek to identify with other groups, like the people at your local gym, in a yoga class, or just a health-conscious group of co-workers? Transferring part of your identity on to a new group takes patience and time, but like the developed skill of healthy eating, it can be accomplished through repetition and exposure. Your first day in a new setting may feel uncomfortable, but remember, if you repeat your effort over several months, your identity will begin to evolve and re-align. *Remember this condition: The pressure to fit into society, relative to food attitudes and body image, was not an issue fifty years ago.* Today, with the number of overweight Americans now in the majority, our culture of excess has evolved into a new 'identity' barrier for those who struggle to lose weight. Are you willing to stand alone and identify with the minority? Can you become a rebel *with* a cause? Accomplish these things and you break down your 'isolation barrier'. If you continue to allow friends and family to influence your eating style, you set yourself up for failure. Make a decision, at this very moment, that your new eating style is acceptable to you. Then, decide, for yourself, that when it comes to your own future health and well-being, *'my personal goal of*

becoming leaner and healthier is far more important than my need to conform.' If you lack confidence in yourself, understanding this barrier and creating a new life goal is a critical step in your path to success. When you reach the point where family and friends label you as 'stubborn', you know you're headed in the right direction. Remember, the culture you live in enables you. You cannot escape or alter this condition. On the other hand, you need to keep your social life intact. When you socialize, begin to offer a more genuine personal benefit – like your willingness to interact with others – instead of offering or indulging in food and drink. Once you separate social eating from social interaction, and once you accept the fact that your new eating style will not be embraced by the majority, you pass through this barrier, and you gain a much clearer vision of how to sustain your effort without the added stress of cultural and social influences.

Barrier Seven: Misunderstanding The Role of Exercise. Exercise is vital for weight management and overall health, but the fact is, it will always play an important 'supporting' role in weight loss. If your current eating habits are poor, using exercise to control your level of body fat is inviting failure. The reality is this: performing a thousand abdominal crunches per week will not result in a 'six pack of well-defined abdominals' without changing the source of your calories and creating a deficit of calories for weeks or months at a time. **Use exercise to improve health, strength, and stamina, but never as a primary solution to weight loss.** Truth is, the hours you spend exercising each week are a fraction of the total hours you spend managing your appetite. In terms of total calories, four hours of exercise accounts for 1,700 to 2,200 additional calories burned per week. For the average adult, however, eating accounts for more than 14,000 calories a week! These numbers define your primary challenge - managing your appetite all day, every day, and attempting to reverse years of poor eating habits.

Don't misunderstand my point here. Exercise is a vital component to weight loss success, but again, media messages (the fitness industry in particular) are often misguided, where the focus on exercise is front and center. If you pay attention to the majority of advertisements, you find product pitch at the forefront, with either a split-second, small print disclaimer referring to 'proper diet' or 'nutritional guide', or, no mention of diet at all. Is this deceptive? You bet. As consumers, we tend to buy into this one dimensional approach, make a purchase, and, two months later, the revolutionary super flex home gym becomes a coat rack. Why? Because you shifted your focus away from identifying and breaking down eating challenges, as well as improving your ability to manage another instinctive fear – ***your resistance to exercise!*** This common misconception – the role exercise plays in weight loss - is a major barrier to success for most Americans. If this is one of your challenges, you only need to perform one simple task. Stop thinking in terms of 'I can exercise my way to an ideal weight' and view your success in terms of 'I will focus on my diet, and use exercise as a catalyst to reach my ideal weight'. Again, when your primary focus is on the creation of new eating habits, this barrier will crumble and no longer block your path to success. Remember, creating a new eating lifestyle is your primary task. Exercise, as important as it is to success, gets an assist.

Barrier Eight: Resistance to Exercise (Exercise Anxiety). Though the process of creating a new eating style takes the lead role in weight loss, exercise is still a critical component to long term success. ***Without exercise, your odds of winning at the diet game fall to one in fifty, if that.*** First and foremost, you need to be aware of your own feelings regarding exercise. For most of us, the thought of forced physical activity provokes anxiety, denial, and often physical discomfort. It becomes a rejected concept, as part of a weight loss plan, because it adds to the stress of calorie deprivation. In order to break through this barrier, whether it's getting started or maintaining a program, you need to know why the thought of exercising causes such a dramatic negative image in your mind. Then, you need to develop a plan that will overcome your subconscious fear of exercise.

First - look at your history regarding exercise. If you fit the profile of the majority, your childhood may have been active, but formal exercise was often controlled by adults. Gym class, team sports, and other activities were scheduled for you and the choice to participate was not yours. As a result, very few adults develop and maintain life-long exercise habits. After High School or College, we are on our own, left to our own devices, and because there are few coaches, teachers, or other role models to mentor or instruct us, we simply fail to establish a routine. We all have an engrained social connection to the rest of humanity, so your tendency is to prioritize the same goals as your family and friends – that is – a focus on career, family, and social life. Very few adult Americans place a high value on exercise because we all tend to identify with a larger group (our culture), and within this group, only a small minority make exercise a priority. The same identity model of behavior applies here, too, because the majority (those who do not exercise) often form a negative opinion of those who do. You hear terms like 'gym rat' or 'health nut' used to describe people who are committed to exercise or health in general. Are these positive terms? Of course not! Remember, it can be emotionally painful to reject traditional roles. It's a very natural progression and re-visiting barrier six, dealing with managing your feelings of isolation, will help here as well. If you step back and look at all your family and friends, you discover that you are not alone in your exercise challenges, and, the answer is yes - there are simple and effective ways to get started and maintain a program.

Though your effort to lose weight will never be shared by everyone in your family and social circle, the need to exercise is universal. For success in developing and maintaining your own plan, three major principles apply.

First – you cannot seclude yourself! Seek help – and pay for it if you have to! Join a gym, a team, a club, or any organization that involves physical activity – even if it's just walking. If you examine success (defined as the ability to sustain a program for a minimum of three years), you see that the odds increase four-fold when you leave the comfort and distractions of your home. If your appearance is a source of anxiety, or, if you feel embarrassed in front of others – get over it! Isn't a poor quality of life or an early death worse? You need to be around others who fit your profile, where you can learn, gain inspiration, and increase the chances of your next exercise plan becoming a lifetime 'habit of choice'.

The second principle is 'compartmentalization'. This term simply means that you set aside a place and time to exercise – you schedule it - and you show up! The common denominator of all successful adults who manage to exercise three to four times a week, year after year, is the 'time and place' label they put on exercising. A famous actor/director once said, "Seventy percent of success is showing up". Though based in sarcasm, this statement is cloaked in truth. All adults can be broken down into two groups when it comes to attitudes regarding exercise. One group 'makes time', or places value in exercise, and the other group rationalizes their lack of intent with 'I don't have the time', 'it's too expensive', or 'I'll start tomorrow' excuses, which, when translated, really means 'I do not place a high value on exercise'. Here is a universal truth about your daily activities: ***You will always find the time to do the things you really want to do.*** It can be tough to admit that you lie to yourself, but if you expect to break down this barrier, you have no choice. If you are not inspired, at this time, to commit to 'showing up', don't beat yourself just yet. Keep reading.

The third principle for success is to set goals that lower your natural resistance. Because of media influence and misconceptions about valid exercise goals, most of us have a problem with developing a strategy that lasts for more than a few weeks or months at a time. Let's shed some light on the truth. ***To minimize both physical and emotional pain, your initial exercise plan has to be simple and minimal.*** As a beginner, beginning brutal 'one-hour-per-day' sessions is a recipe for failure. If you haven't exercised in years, the best plan is that of a moderate routine – like walking, yoga, swimming, biking – perhaps building up to thirty minutes – every other day or twice weekly. If you employ a coach or personal trainer, and they push you hard from day one, fire them immediately and go somewhere else! Many trainers, coaches, and fitness instructors carry false beliefs, and the 'more is better' philosophy of exercise is one of them. For a beginner, long, intense workouts create an overwhelming urge to end the feelings of pain, soreness, and emotional confrontation. And, because these feelings can last for weeks at a time, quitting often becomes a natural event. Most of us make matters worse by recording it as another failure on our life's resume, developing a repetitive pattern of starting and quitting, and the problem becomes worse because failure is now a conditioned, expected outcome. A conservative approach allows you to sustain your effort for months at a time because your anxiety levels are lower. It's a very simple process. The more time you invest, the better your chances. It may take six weeks to gain a comfort level, or it may take six months. Either way, through repetition of moderate routines, you side step the demands of your destructive inner voice (I hate exercising!) and put yourself in a position to form lasting habits.

A note on setting goals and establishing new exercise habits: Remember, most adults have no pre-formed habits for exercise, so if you fit this category, your initial goal is to develop a new habit. The subconscious dynamic is identical to cutting back on calories – repeated conscious efforts eventually migrate into your subconscious and become new behaviors – but remember, this process takes time. Knowing this, it becomes just as important to commit to six months or more with your exercise goals. If you are a beginner, establish two or three sessions per week, 30-45 minutes in length. If you become consistent over a period of six months, you can begin to expand in small increments. Bottom line – exercise should be fun! You need to reach a point in time when you look forward to exercise and the endorphin release it provides. But this won't happen overnight. Remember, too, that exercising three times per week (every other day) can get you into great shape. If you choose to exercise every day, make sure you are fully recovered and energized for each session.

Now that you understand the true relationship of diet and exercise, you need only commit to these three steps to managing a new exercise style. Remember, time is the critical component, so set a goal of six months to a year, where existing anxieties can be transformed into new passions.

Barrier Nine: Resistance to Change. An important mechanism of the human subconscious that most of us never identify is our resistance to change – whether positive or negative in nature. Resistance plays a role in every eating trigger and every behavior you have developed. In essence, your lower brain's desire is to resist all influence – good or bad, because you are, in fact, a creature of habit. ***We are all born with an instinctive fear of change.*** Remember, pleasure and pain are the two primal conditions influencing your behavior, so your tendency is to remain in a comfortable emotional 'zone' where past experiences are known. Eating evolves into a comforting, habitual process because it reduces the pain of hunger and produces feelings of pleasure (endorphins). In the process of replacing your food fix, you have no choice but to venture out of your current emotional zone of comfort. Dieters who succeed do so because they intentionally make themselves uncomfortable through 'forced change', and what separates them from unsuccessful dieters is their drive to sustain the effort for months at a time. Stress levels begin to decrease and the daily decrease in sugar and fat calories is now an evolved, partly subconscious and comfortable habit. This investment of time is the critical component to your success. There is absolutely no way to 'cheat' this process, so understand that these dues must be paid if your goal is to extend beyond the short term and achieve real success.

Because of your natural resistance, changes in eating style have to be maintained for months at a time. There has to be a migration from 'anxious and uncomfortable' feelings to the 'expected and comfortable' state of mind, but this migration can take months – or even years – in many cases. Keep in mind, too, that a major overhaul in your daily lifestyle is a major source of pain, so long term success is next to impossible. The changes you initiate have to be both subtle and consistent to allow for a minimum of anxiety and pain for months at a time. ***Minor changes in your eating behavior allow you to minimize your 'automatic resistance' to change.*** Remember - your subconscious mind will always project a negative outcome when you venture into new territory, so you first have to understand that your instincts, though real, are not essential for your survival in modern times. Second, you have to work around your resistance through the action of subtle change. If you remain defiant and close-minded about this process, you set yourself up to fail. You need to understand the relationship of this barrier with your personal weight loss and exercise challenges. Your 'natural resistance to change' is the foundation on which all weight loss barriers stand. It is a condition that will never be eliminated from your thinking. However, if you understand 'why' you do the things you do, you will have more success through the actions you take to facilitate change.

Barrier Ten: Inspiration vs. Motivation. We all place limits on what we are willing to endure emotionally and physically, so when an emotional line is crossed, the pain of change (beginning a diet, for example) becomes less painful than remaining where you are now (overweight). The result is – you take action! However, when a diet reaches the point of true success, the decision to begin originates out of a personal, evolving emotional conflict, not as a result of being tormented, influenced, embarrassed, ridiculed, or 'instructed' by others. Success is about inspiration, not motivational stimuli. Simply put, inspiration originates from within, and motivation is external - the 'process of being influenced by others'. *Those who consistently fail to lose weight tend to seek out external sources of motivation – a better diet plan, a better exercise routine, or people and environments that will 'motivate' them. For permanent success, however, the decision-making process must originate from personal inspiration, not from the influence of your environment.* Use outside influences and role models to gain inspiration, but do not confuse 'motivating influences' with personal inspiration. They are two separate emotional states. For example, if you hire a personal trainer, and six months later you still rely on their direction and motivation, you simply are not inspired. When inspired, you take the initiative to learn when the situation presents itself. By the sixth month, if you are truly inspired, you know what to do and how to do it. If your personal trainer went on holiday for two weeks and left you on your own, what would make you exercise during that time? Would you know what to do? Inspiration carries you beyond the influence of your experiences, and perpetuates new habits – related to both eating and exercising. The truth is, if you continue to rely on outside centers of influence, you are in trouble! Once you understand the difference and begin to gain inspiration on a personal level, developing a plan and setting goals simply become a 'next step' for you – and your own set of barriers become much easier to manage. Bottom line, you need to know the difference between what motivates you and what inspires you. All successful dieters reach an emotional point of no return - where their own personal threshold of humiliation, negative self- imaging, health issues, ridicule from others, whatever.... forced them to cross an emotional line in the sand and begin to take action. But crossing the line does not guarantee long term success. The lesson here is - if you look to your surroundings for a solution that will influence you, you will fail. If you take what is provided by your environment and use it as a source of personal inspiration, you will succeed. You have to experience your own 'tipping point' and stop expecting others to sell you on the concept of a lean and healthy lifestyle. The fact is, these external sources of motivation - hiring the best personal trainer in town, purchasing a membership in a popular weight loss program, attempting to please your spouse, or simply wishing to impress others at an up-coming social event, are scenarios that spell failure for one simple reason - they all have an ending date!

When you examine the motivators behind a decision to make food sacrifices - never expect consistency. And, do not expect motivation to be contagious. It is not! Not in the world of weight management. Remember, most of your family, friends, and co-workers reject the concept of altering their eating style! The truth is, you have to find your own rationale (why lose weight?) if you want a lifetime conviction to take hold. You must act as your own salesperson, closing a long-term, binding contract with yourself. To help you increase your own level of inspiration, try listing all the positives that come with a lean and healthy lifestyle. Then, write down all the negatives- including the health risks. Finally, compare the two lists. The emotional effect of this exercise alone should help you gain inspiration. Ask yourself the important questions - Are you beginning your diet for the right reason? Are you willing to take on all barriers and commit to a six-month plan? ***Do you have a vision of yourself three years from now, or is the jury still out?*** The information in this book is useless if you remain fixated on temporary goals or the media's 'flavor of the week' diet plan. Keep in mind, too, that you have to perform these painful changes in a somewhat hostile environment, all the while attempting to create a new eating style in direct conflict with your instincts. ***The 'cure', if there is a single solution to reversing weight gain, is defined by the <u>reason</u> you decide to take action, not by the action itself.***

A FINAL NOTE ON BREAKING DOWN BARRIERS

Once you identify and begin to manage the challenges that apply to you, you put yourself in a position to reach your ideal weight and remain there for life. When you find yourself off-track, and you will, review the ten barriers again. They will re-identify your personal challenges and clarify the actions needed to move forward with a winning attitude.

ACHIEVING YOUR GOALS – ONE WEEK AT A TIME

Remember, 1-2 pounds of body fat loss per week is the only legitimate goal you should consider. First, decide the total number of pounds you wish to lose. Then, divide that amount by your 1.5 pound per week goal (as an example), and that will give you a time frame – in the number of weeks required to reach your ideal weight. Forget about the total number when you begin, and focus on the up-coming week's plan of action. Remember, you will always need an escape valve to manage social eating and personal cravings, so plan the week accordingly. Try 18 well-balanced healthy meals, between 400 and 650* calories, as a consistent weekly goal. With some exercise, this should leave you with a few opportunities to indulge. If you are planning a vacation, going through a period of high stress, or simply put in a position where you have little control over your food environment – adjust your goal to 'zero' or accept even a small gain for the up-coming week. Remember - a few 'off-weeks' over the course of a year do not make you a failure! Understand, too, that the longer you sustain your weekly plan of action, the less stressful your new eating lifestyle becomes. *For success, use three simple steps. First, write down your goals and break them down into conservative, weekly objectives! Second, commit to a minimum of six months with both a diet and exercise plan. And finally, make allowances for your human side.* A structured, week by week approach, with conservative 'mini-goals' is your best approach. It helps you cope with the constant stress you feel in first few weeks of your diet. You need escape valves too, because you cannot predict with certainty where and when your resistance might be challenged. Try eating moderate, healthy meals at least 80% of the time (8 out of 10 meals), leaving you some wiggle room for cravings and social eating opportunities. Once you reach your ideal weight, you can then relax your eating style for maintenance of your new body weight. Develop your own style! Before you begin your plan, you must…

*Meal sizes (total calories) will vary according to gender, age, current body weight, and activity levels.

...Establish Control of Your Environment. Purge your kitchen and any other environment you can control. Trash the junk food and begin replacing it with healthy choices for the up-coming week. No cooking oils, other than safflower or olive oil, to be used in small quantities. Dump the deep fryer and convert to the baking or grilling of lean meats and fresh vegetables. No processed carbohydrates – chips, white bread, white rice, or pasta (try whole wheat pasta, bread, whole grain crackers, and brown rice). No high-fat dairy products – butter, whole milk, or cheese. Try alternatives like low-fat margarines, skim milk and yogurt. No processed sugar – cookies, candy, pastries, or soft drinks. Use light mayonnaise, dressings, and other light condiment alternatives. Get in the habit of reading food labels so you can make smart shopping decisions and re-affirm your weekly goal of healthy eating. Plan the purchase of junk foods and poor meal choices accordingly. *Develop a simple standard for purchasing food. For example, a 'Ten percent Rule', where ten percent of your food budget is limited to poor food choices.* Don't test your resolve anymore than you have to – never make poor food purchases with the intent

of indulging several days later. If you are hosting a Sunday 'cookout' or family gathering that includes an abundance of food (they always do), do your grocery shopping on the same day or the day before. In other words, ***why test your resistance if you don't have to?***

Your Duty as a Parent. If you are a parent, environmental control is a must! Remember one important fact about providing food for your children. There is no correlation between love, being a caring parent or good provider, and giving a child what they want when it comes to food. Once the chips, cookies, and candy are vacant from the pantry, you may be scorned as an unfit mother or father, but in reality, the opposite is true. ***As a parent, you should never equate food with love. Providing food as a reward is fine, but it should play only a minor role in the reward system you use.*** Don't scrap the birthday cake or Halloween candy, but understand that children have the same eating instincts as adults. Because children have less impulse control, it becomes the parent's responsibility to control the food environment and the food education of a child. As a parent, you guide your child's life – teaching right and wrong, social skills, and other life lessons, so why not do the same with food and exercise beliefs? Remember, children mimic their parents' behavior, and that includes eating and snacking. If you are overweight, why would you expect your child not to be? If you rarely exercise, place little value on exercise, or fail to promote physical activity, why would your child develop these beliefs on their own? The answer, of course, is that they rarely do. The fact is, children reflect the behavior and attitudes of their parents. The 'lead by example' concept of child-rearing cannot be emphasized enough. But you have to take it a step further.

You have to educate your child. As an adult, if you gain can break away from the status quo, become educated on the basics of nutrition and exercise, you can begin to get your own eating lifestyle together. Once this happens, your children will understand and adapt. As a parent, you prepare your children for life, so education becomes critical. Then - walk the walk – because children emulate what they see in the adult world.

The Real Cause of Childhood Obesity: Childhood obesity is at epidemic levels in America, but contrary to popular belief, the solution is not as simple as educating and motivating children. Children are a direct by-product of our adult culture. We know that children emulate the adult world they live in. They are not born food addicted and lazy. Food and snack advertisements are often directed at children, but ultimately, parents choose the direction – whether it's healthy or poor food choices. Again, look at the skewed, built-in mindset we all have – that if you limit the amount of junk food in your kitchen, you purposely cause pain to your offspring, and therefore, you are a bad parent. Another condition concerning children's behavior is: If the child's parents are overweight, and most of the child's teachers and other adult mentors are overweight, then 'talking the talk' is ineffective. Children learn through observation and tend to ignore communication that conflicts with what they observe. The reality is, once the adult obesity problem in America is resolved, childhood obesity rates will fall by default.

Eating on the Road. When dining out, if you decide to eat healthy, always over-estimate your total calories. When you decide to eat for pleasure, ***enjoy it, then, forget it!*** Remember, as long as you keep your balance of meals intact for the week, you can still reach your goal. At home or work, try surrounding yourself with reminders – written goals, photographs, health and fitness magazines, or even a pair of 'skinny jeans' hanging in plain view. Remember, you have a biological drive to eat when food is available. The daily bombardment of sensory reminders – food and snack commercials, alluring signs on the highway, and the aromas of restaurants and bakeries - can be overwhelming. Avoid environments that put you in harm's way, unless it's part of a planned indulgence.

...Know Your Calorie Set Point'. The FDA has established a daily average of 2,000 calories per day for adults(*). You may burn more or less, but if you are a mature adult (over forty), you should fall close to this average. Keep in mind that this figure is an average, where young adults may require more calories per day, and the elderly (over 65), require less. Because exercise can vary in intensity, using an 'average' of calories burned is the best way to estimate your own daily needs. Using an average of 450 calories burned during one hour of exercise, you would then add 64 calories to your daily average for each hour of intense exercise per week [9]. For example, if you estimate your calorie set point at 2,000 calories per day, and you exercise vigorously twice each week for one hour (total of 900 additional calories burned), your daily set point increases to 2,128 calories. This is the amount of daily calories your body needs to maintain your current weight. Remember, you need a deficit of 3,500 calories to lose one pound of body fat. This translates to a 500 calorie deficit per day – through both an increase in activity and a decrease in food calories – in order to lose one pound of body fat in a week. Purchase a calorie count guide if you need help estimating total calories. Then...

(*) 5, ibid.

........SELECT A NUTRITIONALLY SOUND DIET THAT YOU CONTROL! It's not difficult to find healthy, low-calorie alternatives at your local grocery - even the pre-packaged variety. Why would you have meals delivered to you? Is your intent to become a social recluse as well? The fact is, the higher your dependency on a structured plan (delivered meals, counseling, etc.), the more you condition yourself to become dependent. Is your life really that structured? Do you eat every meal or snack in the solitude of your home? If so, are you willing to forgo any social events that may involve food, or, can you even commit to such a rigid lifestyle (not to mention the money) for ten years? Twenty years? Remember, in the real world, if long term success is your desired outcome, you need to allow for flexible goals. You also need to take complete responsibility for the food you eat. It is not difficult (and not as expensive) to purchase healthy alternatives at your local market. If you can't find the time, or you have the money to burn, you're admitting to a half-hearted effort, because, in reality, you will always find the time to do what you really want to do. If you need a list of recommended foods or recipes, there are hundreds of diet books on the market promoting nutritionally sound plans. Like choosing a tool for a specific task, you need only to pick one. Bottom line, choosing a well balanced, natural diet, low in saturated fats, refined sugars, and void of processing, translates into a simple shopping agenda, easily supported by your local grocery, and easy to put into place.

Setting Exercise Goals. If you are not exercising now, make only moderate changes that reduce the pain of confrontation with starting an exercise program. Try 30 minutes of a low impact activity, like walking, swimming, or biking, three times a week. After 4-6 weeks, expand your routine in small increments. If you are exercising now, try a small increase – ten added minutes of training per workout. To reduce the anxiety that comes with starting or maintaining an exercise routine, don't go it alone! Join a friend, a group, a team, a club, or a gym, where you can identify and gain inspiration. It's important to reach the six-month mark, where you begin to view exercise as a habit of choice rather than an unpleasant chore.

WEIGHT MANAGEMENT AND AGING

There is a single fact you need to be aware of as you approach middle age (50). For both men and women, hormone levels decrease over time, and because hormone levels have a direct influence on muscle and bone mass, your metabolic rate decreases with age. It's a natural part of the human aging process. For this reason, when you reach a mature age, your daily calorie requirements are lower, and, with the loss of muscle mass and bone density, your calorie needs may fall even further. You have to make adjustments as you age, but there are ways to help you minimize this effect.

The closest thing you will ever find to the 'fountain of youth' is a three-pronged approach to living your life. First, as you age, you need to keep your body fat levels low and your diet healthy. The more you avoid processed sugars, starches, high fat foods, and an excess of calories, the slower your body will age. You must also avoid de-hydration and exposure to toxins like tobacco, alcohol, drugs, chemicals added to foods and beverages, and, contaminated air and water. *Second,* you need to manage stress. Once you understand stress (covered in barrier four), you can take steps to reduce the destructive effects on your own body and mind. The expression 'Don't worry – be happy' applies here. Your stress levels will remain high if you fail to understand and accept your inability to control the world you live in. The negative emotions associated with stress– anxiety, fear, depression, worry – contribute to chronic stress and fatigue. These emotional states are accelerators in the aging process. *Finally,* you need to exercise. Any form of exercise is good, but resistance training is best. No need to become a hardcore 'weightlifter', but some form of training is needed to keep your muscle mass intact, your bones dense, and your hormone levels high. Research has proven that, for both men and women, just one hour of resistance training per week increases muscle mass, bone density, and hormone levels[10]. If you embrace these three simple principles and make them part of your life, you can enhance your own quality of life – well into your senior years.

Keep this condition in mind, too. When we are young, our bodies can tolerate added body fat resulting from a poor diet, a sedentary lifestyle, or both. But this lifestyle cannot continue into adulthood and middle age without health consequences. As a middle-aged adult, carrying forty extra pounds (or more), with little exercise, is a recipe for disaster. In fact, for health reasons, the older you become, the more you need to lower body fat levels and remain active. With a fifty year-old heart, lungs, and circulatory system (not to mention the other organs), added body fat becomes much more of a burden on middle aged adults.

What is a healthy percentage of body fat for adult men and women? ***Most physicians recommend 11-15% for men and 15-20% for women.***[11] Bottom line, when you reach a mature age, you need to take the extra work load off your body. It marks the difference between those who maintain a high quality of life well into old age and those who end up with health issues and a fully stocked medicine cabinet. The reality is, when you examine your own health, the combination of a poor diet, high levels of stress, and a sedentary lifestyle are the 'big three' in age acceleration.

MYTH VERSUS FACT

Continue Your Education! With so many false beliefs about nutrition, weight loss, and exercise, it becomes essential for your success to know the facts. Here are six common myths you need to be aware of:

Myth 1: The more meals you skip, the faster you lose weight.
Truth: Skipping meals is counterproductive to weight loss because it adversely affects your metabolic rate and your body chemistry. Starving yourself will force your body into a 'survival mode', ready to replenish glycogen levels (blood sugar) and store body fat as soon as you begin eating again. In addition, advanced stages of hunger have a destructive effect on your cravings – you seek the most calorie-dense foods (high in fats, sugars, etc.) in order to gain energy quickly – all bad news for you. A daily habit of eating healthy, low calorie, well-balanced meals every 4-5 hours is the most effective long-term method of weight loss.

Myth 2: Food consumed at night will be stored as body fat.
Truth: Only excess calories above your daily set point are stored as body fat. Even if most of your calories are consumed in the evening, you cannot gain weight unless your daily total is above your set point. For example, if your late night snacking adds 800 calories to the 1,000 calories you have consumed that day, you will continue to lose weight if your body's daily calorie requirement is close to the adult average of 2000. Think 'total daily calories'.

Myth 3: You can target or 'spot reduce' body fat.

Truth: Biologically, the human body breaks down fat in a pre-disposed manner, with genetics playing the key role in the location of where and how fat cells are accumulated or eliminated. In women, hips and thighs are often the last place where body fat is noticeably lost, even after months of dieting. In men, it may be the lower abdominal fat that's the last to go. A thousand stomach crunches per week may burn added calories and firm up your mid-section, but the sub-dermal fat in your abdomen, the visceral fat around your internal organs, and other fat cells within your body cannot be isolated for the purpose of reduction through diet or exercise.

Myth 4: Aerobics is the most effective exercise for losing body fat.
Truth: Resistance Training is the single most effective exercise for lowering body fat. The biological truth is - lean muscle cells require more nourishment and energy (calories) to maintain than fat cells. Adding only one pound of lean muscle through resistance exercise increases the number of calories you burn per hour, even when you are at rest. Aerobic activity burns calories, but it has two pitfalls. It has little influence on your resting metabolic rate, and, in addition to burning body fat as fuel, it reduces muscle mass! Resistance training maintains your lean mass and increases your rate of calorie burn twenty four-seven…. even when you sleep! The winner – resistance training!

Myth 5: Drugs, herbs, and other supplements are essential for effective weight loss.
Truth: The simple answer is 'supplements are not necessary'. Weight loss will always be a two step process. First, you have to identify your personal triggers and develop a plan of action

to manage them. You have to commit – for several months – to your effort. Finally, you choose your support tool - a well-balanced nutrition plan to follow. Natural supplements, food alternatives – even chemical inhibitors - are secondary tools of the trade, to be put in place once control is established. Taking stimulants in order to suppress your appetite without any attempt to change your eating style is working in reverse, because your personal barriers are masked temporarily. Start with an approach where you identify and manage your own set of obstacles. Then, you can use natural, herbal remedies, always in moderation, as a secondary tool.

Myth 6: It takes thirty days to change eating habits.
Truth: Habits are formed through both conscious and subconscious intent. A cognitive, or conscious habit, like brushing your teeth in the morning, can certainly be formed over a period of thirty days, but altering habits developed through lower brain instincts are much more challenging, and they include your primitive drive to eat. For change to occur, your resistance to ancient eating impulses has to improve, and this simply won't happen without several months of repeated effort. Remember, you develop coping skills through repetition. Thirty days is enough for temporary success, but it's not enough time for new behaviors to evolve into habits of choice. If you love ice cream, for example, and you eliminated ice cream from your diet for thirty days, would you still have the desire for ice cream? Of course you will. The drive is always there, so eliminating the foods you enjoy is not a practical solution. What you can do, however, is make small sacrifices over a period of several months – perhaps two servings of ice cream per week instead of five. Thirty days later, the sacrifice remains stressful and

confrontational. At sixty days, it's still somewhat of a challenge. However, after six months of two servings of ice cream per week, you develop a new pattern of eating that lacks the emotional conflict of the first month. At the one year mark, your conscious intent evolves into subconscious habit, and five servings of ice cream per week is now a distant, non-confrontational memory. As a result, the destructive inner voice you heard in the first month is now barely a whisper. Maintaining your new body, void of the twenty pounds you carried a year ago, is a new, subconscious desire. The result is, the choice to 'overindulge' becomes more confrontational than the sacrifices needed to stay lean, so these small sacrifices become your new standard of thinking. This is how you establish new and improved eating habits. If you are having trouble accepting or understanding this process, re-read barrier three – Developing Resistance Skills.

NUTRITIONAL TIPS THAT WORK

1. ***Lean protein is essential!*** Proteins from animal or vegetable sources help you feel full for longer periods than do fats or processed carbohydrates. Develop the habit of eating lean protein with every meal.

2. ***Drink water!*** Six to eight glasses of water a day is sound advice. Try drinking water with your meals instead of soft drinks, tea, coffee, juices, or diet beverages.

3. ***Eat fiber!*** Twenty to twenty five grams each day. Fiber-rich foods, such as whole grains, fresh vegetables, and fruits allow for a larger volume of food with fewer total calories. Your stomach registers volume, not calories, when signaling your brain that you are 'full', so a fiber-rich diet is essential for weight loss. As an added benefit, 25 grams of fiber consumed each day will help you maintain excellent digestive health.

4. ***Be conscious of your energy needs.*** Try to consume most of your carbohydrate calories early in the day, preferably for breakfast and lunch. Afternoon fatigue is often the result of a lack of available carbohydrate energy. Look at carbohydrates (both complex and simple) as energy sources. Most adults have a much lower expenditure of energy in the evening, so a daily descending carbohydrate style of eating is best.

5. ***Eat a healthy breakfast!*** A low-fat, high protein breakfast with natural carbohydrate sources re-affirms your focus, creates healthy insulin levels after several hours of sleep, and gives you a positive mindset for the rest of the day. When you break from your plan early, you are more likely to go off-track with the rest of your meals that day. It's a mind game you can't win, so keep breakfast healthy. If you plan to eat a decadent meal or snack, make it a mid-day or evening event.

6. ***Don't 'Eat on the Run'.*** Sit down, relax, and eat meals slowly and without distractions. When you finish, leave the table immediately! People who 'compartmentalize' eating (intentionally set aside a time and place for meals), have a much greater chance for long term weight loss success.

7. ***The lemon-lime effect.*** Try an eight ounce glass of lemon or lime juice concentrate mixed with four parts water thirty minutes before mealtime (add honey or artificial sweetener if you can't handle the bitter taste). It reduces your level of hunger and aides in digestion as well. Acidic juices also help with recovery from vigorous exercise, helping your system remove blood toxins, including lactic acid, and bringing you back into a normal ph range, where recovery is accelerated.[12]

EXERCISE TIPS THAT WORK

1. *Cycle your carbohydrates*! Carbohydrates are your body's preferred source of energy. Though proteins and fats can be converted into energy, simple and complex carbohydrates are a direct fuel source for your body's engine. Think of proteins and fats as crude oil, which has to be converted into fuel before it can become a source of energy. The two forms of exercise, aerobic and anaerobic, translate into two 'best methods' of carbohydrate consumption. You need carbohydrate calories for anaerobic activity, but total carbohydrate calories should be limited before aerobic activity for best results. The reason is simple. For effective anaerobic training, especially with resistance exercise, carbohydrates provide the energy needed for an effective workout and maintenance of your lean muscle mass. With aerobic exercise, however, your intent, in addition to cardiovascular and conditioning benefits, is to reduce body fat. To do this effectively, pre-workout carbohydrate and fat calories should be restricted to help your body reduce glycogen levels and convert to the burning of body fat as a source of fuel. Protein should never be restricted. Think of carbohydrate calories as 'fuel calories'.

2. *Recuperate from your workouts!* Allow your body the time it needs to recover from exercise. More is not always better. Both the intensity and the length of each workout demand recuperation

time. Exercising every other day can still get you into great shape and assist you with your weight loss plan. Don't fall into the 'You should exercise every day' belief. It's simply not true.

3. ***Running is not a necessity!*** A 35 minute brisk walk is more effective in burning body fat than a 10 minute jog (slow run). And, for heart and lung health, fast-paced walking can be just as effective. If you are more than thirty pounds overweight, running may also compromise your bones, joints, and tendons with undue stress. Unless you are training for a running event or competition (or simply prefer running), try fast-paced walking instead. For best results (loss of body fat), try 35 to 45 minutes, or two to four miles in distance, at least twice each week, or the equivalent time on an elliptical, stair-master, bike, or 'low-impact' swimming. Again, glycogen levels (blood sugar from food sources) will determine whether or not you tap into your body fat reserves. If your liver and muscles are chalk-full of glycogen from a recent overindulgence, expect only minor success. For optimum results, eat a small, high protein, low calorie meal or snack an hour before aerobic exercise. Force your body to go after fat reserves as a source of fuel. Take your focus off the 'hard and fast' approach to aerobic training.

4. ***Avoid heavy meals before exercise.*** Heavy, calorie dense, high fat meals require a concentrated effort by your digestive tract. With added blood flow to the stomach and intestines, you will often

experience sluggishness and fatigue (Thanksgiving dinner is a prime example). The result is: you lose your inspiration to exercise. If you plan on eating a large meal, make it a 'post-exercise' experience.

5. ***Don't go it alone!*** Join a team, a class, a group, or a gym to help you establish long-term exercise habits. Surveys show a long-term success rate of 20% for adults who commit to a gym or other forms of group exercise. Success rates fall to 5% for those who try the 'do-it-yourself' approach at home. You are four times more likely to develop long-term exercise habits if you leave the comfort and distractions of home.[13]

BREAKING DOWN BARRIERS – A REVIEW

1. ***Educate yourself!*** It's an easy challenge to overcome, but it's a major indicator of your intent and level of inspiration.

2. ***Get a Life!*** There's a lot more to life than the joy of eating. To conquer food addiction challenges, expand other passions, especially the physical ones, and addictive food behaviors can be kept in check.

3. ***Develop the skill of healthy eating.*** There are no shortcuts – commit to your new eating style for a minimum of six months and it becomes second nature – for life!

4. ***Get a handle on stress.*** Control what you can, and forget about the rest. Remember – dieting is an added form of stress! Start investing in yourself – with more downtime and rest.

5. ***Accept your human side.*** Going off-track is a given. Plan for indulgences and the feelings of guilt are gone, along with your desire to give up and return to old habits.

6. ***Be willing to 'go it alone'.*** When support is offered, take it, but never expect consistent support when you intentionally separate yourself from the social influence of eating.

7. **Understand the relationship between diet and exercise**, so you know where to put most of your focus. Managing your impulse to eat is a twenty-four seven effort. Exercise is vital, but it will always play a supporting role in weight loss.

8. *Get started with some form of moderate exercise!* Remember, the goals you set need to be in writing, and they need to allow for small, incremental changes that reduce your resistance. If you are a beginner, set aside a time and place to exercise outside the distracting environment of your home.

9. *Win the battle with your subconscious!* When you understand your built-in resistance to change, you learn how to overcome forced sacrifices (pain) with incremental changes. Remember, habits begin as a learned conscious behavior, slowly evolving in the subconscious over time. New eating behaviors are no different!

10. *Diet for the right reason!* What's driving you to change? If people or events motivate you to act, your efforts are likely to be temporary. If you are inspired and begin your plan without the concept of an ending date, you put yourself in a position to succeed.

FINALLY

The single most important commodity you will ever own is your health. Yet, in our culture, social status, achievement, and success are often measured in the value of our accumulated wealth and assets, instead of the condition of our bodies and minds. The point I make here is this: Too many adults look back on their life, as they lay dying in a hospital bed from complications brought on by a lifetime of over-eating and under-exercising, and have this epiphany; 'I wish I had taken better care of myself'. The decision you need to make now is just as serious.

With a solid understanding of a 'back door' approach to changing eating behavior, you can apply what you have learned and reverse your history of weight gain. Your challenges may be specific to you, but the barriers you need to break down are universal, so take comfort in the fact that you are not alone. Work on your own plan of action. Remember, a major lifestyle overhaul is often ineffective. Make subtle changes you can tolerate over the long haul. Then, within your plan, make allowances for some wiggle room. ***Write down your goals, be conservative in your approach, and, most important, be patient.*** Decades of poor habits cannot be managed inside of a few weeks. It will take six months to a year for most of you to reverse the path you are on, and if you cannot accept this future, you will always be a victim of the 'weight loss blues'. Some confrontation is needed, too. Exercise provokes anxiety and resistance, so you may need to punch through this psychological wall as well. You may have to confront many of your beliefs and reject most of what you see and hear in the media. You may need to wipe your educational slate clean and start from scratch. Most of the answers you need are within the pages of this book. To help sustain your effort, re-read the barriers that apply to you. Weight loss challenges, like a fingerprint, are unique for each of us, so you need to develop a plan based on your own set of obstacles and stop relying on advice from outside sources, unless their recommendations are based on the same approach. Remember, if you remain passive and continue to wait for the right moment to make a decision, it may be years before an 'inspirational event' comes along. Become active, and begin to seek out personal sources of inspiration on a daily basis. And most important, start today!

Now that you understand how your drive to eat works against you, you can take action and begin to make progress. Once your plan is in place, examine the 'reason' you chose to begin, because your rationale for taking action is just as important. Your level of inspiration may not be where it needs to be at this moment in time. But there is good news. Inspiration will develop and grow over time, and, to your advantage, your level of knowledge is far more advanced at this time.

The truth is, we all have life goals and daily intentions that are unrelated to eating. You need to tap into these other agendas and allow them to replace the addictive allure of your favorite foods and snacks. The question you have to ask yourself is: 'Am I inspired enough – at this time - to take action?'

The magic bullet, for you, is a willingness to identify your own set of obstacles, take some form of action to manage them, and understand that, for true success, you have to follow the beat of your own drum, ignore virtually all media messages, and commit to the time.

The thirty second response to the question of: 'how do I lose weight and keep it off?' is simple and straight forward: **FORGET ABOUT SPEED (HOW SOON CAN I REACH MY IDEAL WEIGHT?). MAKE SMALL SACRIFICES YOU CAN TOLERATE FOR A MINIMUM OF SIX MONTHS. THEN, ALLOW FOR SOME INDULGENCES. THIS ONE ACTION ALONE WILL TRIPLE YOUR CHANCE OF SUCCESS.** (Remember, success is defined by your ability to reach an ideal weight and remain there for three years.)

Keep an open mind and refer to guidelines in this book on a regular basis. Bottom line – you can change your life!

ENDNOTES

1   Published Statistics, Center for Disease Control and Prevention, 2013.

2   Diet Review Post, 2013. Success as defined by the ability to maintain weight loss, within 2% of an original goal weight over a period of 3 years.

3   Published findings, Center for Disease Control and Prevention, 2012

4   Published Data, Food and Drug Administration, 2010

5   Adult average daily calorie requirement as established by the Food and Drug Administration

6   Published Study, Current Biology, September, 2013.

7   Staff Article, Mayo Clinic, 'Stress symptoms: Effects on Your Body and Behavior', 2012.

8   Published Findings, Journal of American Medical Association (JAMA), Internal Medicine Archives, 'Sleep Disturbance and Obesity', 2001.

9   Web MD, published article, 2012

10 Published Study, American Physiological Society, 'Effects of Heavy Resistance Training on Hormonal Response Patterns', April, 1999.

11 Published Recommendations for Body Fat Percentages, World Health Organization, National Institute of Health, 2000.

12 Published Benefits of Lemon Juice, themedicalquestions.com, 'How Do I Get Rid of Lactic Acid?', 2013.

13 *Results based on a survey of 1,450 adults, maintaining a gym-based exercise program versus an 'at-home' program, for a minimum of two years, conducted by Wave Cyle Systems, LLC, 2011.*

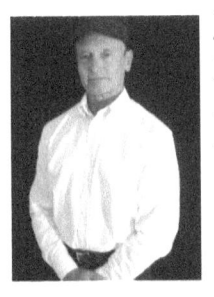**Jim Cabeceiras** is one of America's premier weight loss authorities and published weight loss authors. He has a background in college athletics, bodybuilding, personal training, and more than thirty years of experience in working with clients in the field of weight management. Through research and consultation with physicians, psychiatrists, nutritionists, and the nation's leading fitness trainers, a backdoor approach to weight management was developed in 2007. How to Beat the Weight Loss Blues is a step-by-step guide that defines this highly successful approach.

www.ingramcontent.com/pod-product-compliance
Lightning Source LLC
Chambersburg PA
CBHW050422290526
45786CB00003B/1367